# Rucking Gains

# Rucking Gains

■ ■ ■

*Josh Bryant and Adam benShea*

# Rucking Gains

JoshStrength, LLC and Adam benShea

Copyright © 2020

# Table of contents

# Introduction

There is a difference between a fountain and a well. A fountain, like that found outside of a Vegas casino or a Palm Springs resort, will spout or shoot water high into the air. It gives the image of bountiful water, certainly desirable for any desert denizen. But, at close inspection, the careful eye will notice that the base of the fountain is shallow and actually holds little liquid. There is not much water there. It is simply an illusion of water wealth.

In contrast, a well is rarely marked by much more than a subtle upwelling. Without the telltale man-made water pulley systems, it can be easy to miss a well. In fact, work in the form of digging is often required to reach the liquid resources buried deep in underground aquifers. However, once a well is found, its bounty may come up from deep down into middle earth and keep providing you with pure water.

A fountain gives a great show. But, if you're looking for nourishment, it would leave you thirsty.

A well is unassuming. Yet, it's full of enriching sustenance.

This analogy works for people. It is also true for gyms.

Many folks shop around for a place to work out like they're window-shopping for the holiday season. They gaze longingly at the shining equipment and the spandex-clad enthusiasts astride the cardio machines. These people get taken in by the glamour and glitter, only to find themselves in an overdressed strip mall chrome palace that lacks the necessary atmosphere and infrastructure for making real gains.

Well, the gym from our high school days was certainly not overdressed. It didn't feature the latest equipment, and many of the lifters wouldn't make the cut for a catwalk fashion show (unless somebody was doing a lumberjack line of flannels or going for the denim long-haul trucker look). It did have lots of iron and the type of atmosphere where hard training was not welcomed, but expected. It wasn't the place where training was sold as a form of materialism. It was the place where you came for gains.

Our gym had real depth. It was a well, not a fountain.

The cast of characters who trained at that weight pile had depth, also.

The casual onlooker could have looked at the gym and seen a bunch of construction workers, strip club bouncers, and ex-jocks.

The seasoned observer would see devotees to the iron. The commitment to training at that place rivaled what you would find at any Nepalese monastic community.

Similarly, where many saw a bunch of hobos lining the streets of old Monterey, John Steinbeck saw a modern round table of Arthurian knights, and he captured their rich exploits in his written work (think *Cannery Row* and *Sweet Thursday*).

The nobility of the characters at our old gym was seemingly bottomless, if you were just willing to dig. We were willing to dig, and listen.

We listened and we learned from Thic Vic (*Tactical Strongman: The Complete Guide*), Old School Frank (*Tactical Density Training*), Al Torrio (*Speed Strong*), Coach Chiefy (*8 x 8 Off-Season Powerlifting Program*), Bosco (*Time under*

*Tension: Tactical Training*), and, of course, Chato (*The Saga of the Tijuana Barbell Club*).

If you are willing to pay attention, life is full of lessons.

Our drive to the gym was scenic, taking us along the picturesque shore of our beachfront community. While we were making the drive one day, our truck was enveloped in the thick mist of an almost tangible marine layer that floated inland from the ocean.

Never interested in letting a pattern dull our sensory awareness, even on a drive we made many times, we paid attention to the happenings on our route. Through the dense fog on the beach, we could just make out a lone figure carrying a backpack and walking at a good clip through the sand.

At first glance, there was nothing particularly special about this individual. In fact, he could have been one of the many flotsam and jetsam types who seem to congregate around beaches the world over.

Never satisfied with a hasty glimpse, we looked closer. There was something distinct about this figure. He walked with a military bearing and moved with a sense of purpose and pride. His stride was quick and powerful. He clearly had a profound kinesiological awareness.

This guy was not just some aimless beach walker. There was more to this man. There was depth.

We both took note, before returning our attention to the drive and getting our minds right for the intense workout ahead of us.

It was a good workout. We brought an intentional mindset to our workout and maintained intensity throughout the duration of the session. On our way out the door and down the ramp to the parking lot, we caught sight of Thic Vic (whose pearls of training wisdom we shared in *Tactical Strongman: The Complete Guide*).

He was engrossed in serious conversation with someone we didn't know, but as we got closer, we recognized him as the guy from the beach.

We gave a subtle wave to Thic Vic as a greeting, not wanting to interrupt their discussion.

Brow furrowed, Thic Vic looked over and gave us a curt nod before turning back to this mystery man.

We were left wondering, who was this guy?

A couple days later we again ran into Thic Vic at the gym, where he was just finishing some dumbbell work.

"Hey fellas, how are things?" he asked when he saw us. Thic Vic took a sincere interest in our training and our lives.

"We're just getting ready to do some interval training. What have you been up to?"

"Well, I've been catching up with an old friend from my time in the service." Thic Vic's military career was the stuff of legend and mystique in our community. "Oh, here he comes now."

A broad-shouldered, lean-hipped, chiseled-featured man with a clear military bearing made his way over.

"Fellas," Thic Vic said, "this is Deano. We're old friends and he's a great guy. But, Deano don't play."

Deano looked at us with a stare that could cut glass.

To hold his gaze, we remembered an old trick our freshman football coach taught us, something he learned during basic training before going to 'Nam. He said that when you meet someone who gives you that thousand-yard stare, a look of raw intensity, don't look away. Stare at their forehead. This will enable you to endure the most intense stare.

After a minute that felt like an eternity, Deano gave us a quick look of approval.

"Thic Vic told me about you guys. He said you train hard. I like that."

Like pulling a knife from a hip sheath, he brought up his hand in one smooth, quick motion. Some men give a limp handshake, while others put every muscle fiber into the action as a means to prove some kind of adolescent masculinity. In the case of Deano, his handshake was tight as a vice grip, but it was machine like. He wasn't trying to prove anything. It was almost like gripping a robot programmed only for strength.

"Thank you," we replied in sincere appreciation for the compliment. Praise like that from Thic Vic was cause for genuine pride in the focus we brought to the gym.

"Hey, were you at the beach the other day? Walking, really fast, through the dense fog?" we asked, letting our youthful curiosity bubble to the surface.

Deano gave an almost imperceptible grin.

"I sure was," he said. "But I was rucking."

"Rucking? What's that?"

"It's walking at a fast clip, with a rucksack, hence the name. It is the foundational activity of any infantry unit from the Roman legionnaires of yesteryear to the great Gurkha rifle regiments of the British army."

"So, you do it because of your time in the military?"

"That's part of it. But, there's more to it. Cardio-wise it's one of the best options out there. Especially, as you age, you carefully choose your workout." Deano gave a slight chuckle before continuing. "I'm no spring chicken, so I need to be careful with my body. I have to take care of my body so I can rely on it when I need it."

It was hard to tell Deano's age. His face was weather-beaten and decorated with a labyrinth of scars, while his military olive colored T-shirt did little to hide a muscular torso that would be the envy of any twenty-something gym goer.

"Could you tell us a little more about rucking?" we asked with sincere curiosity and interest.

"You know, boys, I will and I'll do you one better. I'll teach you how to use it in your workouts."

Like the man, the workout Deano shared with us was short on flash but deep in depth. We listened intently as he explained the simple beauty of rucking.

# Chapter I

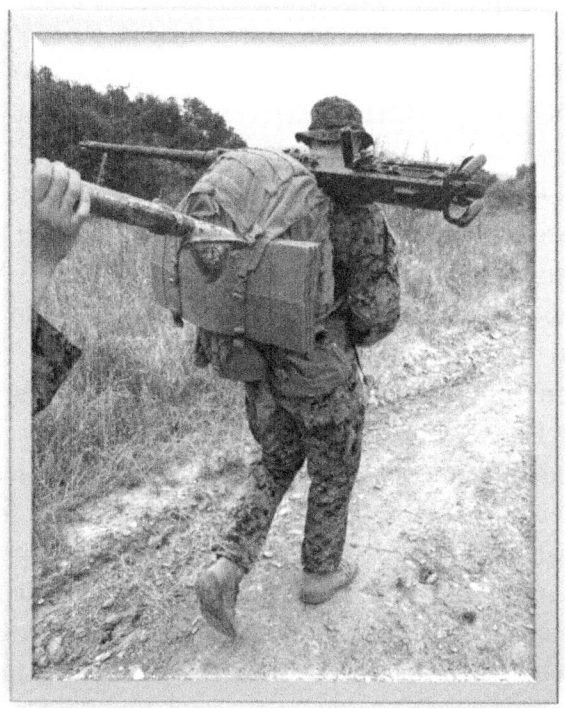

**Figure 1. Harry Walker rucking in South Africa.**

In its original definition, rucking is walking with intention with weight in a rucksack/backpack. Since then, it's evolved into the definition we will be using: a relatively fast walk over distance carrying a load, commonly now including a weighted vest.

A core military skill for infantry units and special forces groups throughout the world, rucking requires strength, endurance, and character—while simultaneously building it.

In fact, rucking may be considered the foundation and standard training for any military land-based unit. From the Roman legion to the French legionnaires, they all ruck.

For reference, here are some rucking standards from armed forces around the world. These will give you a sense of different rucking protocols, which can be used for goal-setting purposes.

**US Armed Forces.** For a candidate to gain the Expert Infantryman Badge (an elite qualification for infantry personnel), candidates must complete a ruck march of 12 miles in three hours or less while carrying a rifle and load. In totality, this can be up to 70 pounds!

**French Legion.** For legionnaires to complete their annual fitness test training, they must complete a five-mile ruck loaded with rifle, helmet, and a 26-pound pack in under 40 minutes and a 16-mile night march in three hours with a 40-pound load. Other marches of longer distances are part of their training, including the "Kepi march" of 31 miles in full combat gear carrying a rifle, helmet, and a 49-pound load and the 62-mile "Raid march" in full combat gear carrying a rifle, helmet, and a 49-pound load over a three-day period while navigating and simulating what goes on in battle.

**British Armed Forces.** In the British Army, rucking is considered a core skill and is tested annually as part of their fitness tests. Soldiers carry 33 to 55 pounds over eight miles, depending on their job, and the test must be completed within three and a half hours. Infantry soldiers are expected to pass even more advanced tests.

## Why Ruck?

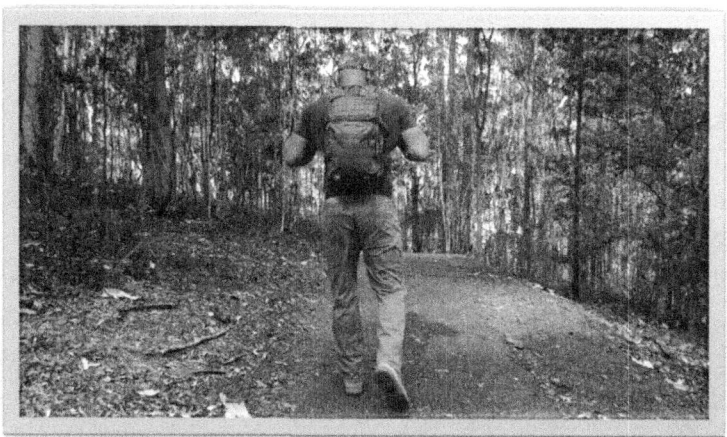

**Figure 2. Tom Haviland rucking in parts unknown.**

Okay, you get it, these soldiers are in amazing physical condition! But you aren't training for war or even a career as a tactical athlete, so should you ruck? And what benefits do you stand to derive?

### Cardio for Cardio Haters

Maybe it was Sergeant Ignacio Coral, the toughest Mexican this side of Pancho Villa, who screamed at you as you jogged while he reeked of 90 proof the morning after one of his legendary benders of fast women, whiskey, and cigars.

Or it may have been your sixth-grade gym teacher, the former "softball great" with the pixie haircut, who forced you to swim laps when you could barely swim.

3

Whatever the reason, we get it—you hate cardio!

We are here to introduce you to rucking, the cardio choice for the cardio haters.

Why rucking? Because rucking offers a myriad of benefits that directly transfer to real life. We are going to take a cursory overview of those benefits.

## Lower Impact

The elliptical is easier on the body than jogging, and not a bad choice if you are 80 years old and dealing with arthritis. But, did you know that rucking is much less stressful on your body than running?

Biomechanical studies on running reveal the tremendous cyclical forces to which the knee is exposed. These forces can be 7 to 11 times your bodyweight! And if your technique is off, the onset of pain will begin even sooner. Contrast that to rucking, which puts two to three times the force of your body-weight onto your knee with each step, and it's easy to see that rucking is simply less taxing on your body.

## Improved Posture

The weight of a backpack pulls your shoulders back and puts you in the right alignment to improve your posture. As you ruck more, your body is being trained to stay in its proper position; it's almost like doing a plank that requires dynamic stability.

## Outdoor Workout

There are myriad scientific studies that show both mental and physical health benefits from being outside. Any doubts, lock yourself in your room and play Dungeons and Dragons for a week and see how you feel. With the COVID quarantines, suicide and nonfatal mental health issues have been on the rise. One way to combat this, without violating stay-at-home orders, is to get outside and ruck! Additionally, you will be showered in nature's best antidepressant, vitamin D from the sun, and experience the great outdoors. Regardless of quarantines, you will feel better psychologically and physically when you get outside in nature.

## Burn More Calories

A 200-pound man who jogs at a 12-minute mile pace for an hour, which is 5.0 MPH, will burn approximately 755 calories. The same person walking quickly at 3.5 MPH will burn 391 calories; adding a ruck to this walk, that same man would burn 50 percent more calories, approaching 600 calories in an hour, and some research indicates the total may be much higher. On the lower end, you are still close to jogging in burning calories, but you are also getting stronger and improving your posture while not running your body into the ground. If you walk every day, just throwing a weight in your backpack or throwing on a weighted vest will add up quickly over the course of weeks, months, and years for fat loss via caloric expenditure.

## Build Strength/Muscle

Jogging excessively rids your body of hard-earned muscle; rucking can build muscle, particularly in your shoulders, core, back, and the elusive, purple unicorn of muscular development, the traps. The traps respond very well to being stretched under load; think farmer's walks. While your load when rucking won't be as heavy as what you'd use when doing farmer's walks, you will be working under a continuous load for 20 minutes or more. If you have never rucked, usually the first area to fatigue is the traps—imagine that, cardio that assists in building a no-nonsense physique.

### Prevent Injury

Assuming you don't overdo it and you follow our programs, you can relieve existing back pain and/or use rucking as a prehab mechanism. As you strengthen your back and core muscles, you also strengthen your hips and posture, making you less likely to get injured in general. All of these muscles must be continuously engaged as your legs keep trekking you forward. As your upper body supports the load, you build tremendous strength endurance, the kind that serves you when the shit hits the fan in a free-for-all tussle at the Bangkok ex-pat bar on dollar sake night.

### Build an Aerobic Base/Conditioning

Rucking improves your readiness and your ability to recover; simply put, it builds your work capacity. Because it elevates your heart rate, it has a similar effect on the heart as jogging, without the documented downsides. Having an aerobic base is important. Besides keeping the ticker healthy, it enables you to recover faster between sets, workouts, sprints, or rounds in a pit fight; basically, training-wise, you can do more, more often, because of the regenerative qualities of your aerobic base. Aerobics does not have to be a dirty word with rucking.

### Minimalist Simplicity

All you need is yourself, a rucking backpack or weighted vest, and a decent pair of shoes.

### Low Cost

Assuming you have a decent pair of shoes, you can easily get started rucking for less than $100. Contrast that to overcrowded, poodle-dick palace commercial gyms that charge twice that for a month's membership.

## Anywhere, Anytime
You can ruck while walking with your kids, with your friends, up and down the stairs in your apartment complex, or on your favorite hiking trail. Or impress your latest Tinder rendezvous with an afternoon of rucking. Rucking is available at all times. Now that lockdowns are on the table, this value cannot be disputed. Don't let your strength and conditioning be at the mercy of the government.

## Training While Travelling
It is tough to pack a bench press or squat rack in a travel bag, but a rucksack is not so difficult. Eight-hour layover in Baghdad? Ruck around the airport or get really ambitious and go out and grab a beef kabob, sightsee, and stay on your rucking routine.

## Functional Fitness
10,000 years ago, hunters didn't have pickup trucks to transport their kills, and farmers in Mesopotamia had to carry their crops. Weighted carries have always been a part of the human experience! We need this ability to survive and thrive.

## Socializing
In his discussion on rucking, Brett McKay of *The Art of Manliness* fame reminds us that man is a social creature. Rucking is something anyone can do, and it's a great idea to invite a friend to join you. There are plenty of ruck groups, and you can easily find one on the website GoRuck.com. So it's great for making friends or finding that alluring romantic partner who likes sweating alongside you.

## Scaling

Unlike a deadlift that requires either stripping off or adding plates to change the difficulty, rucking is very easily scalable. If your rucking workout is too easy, find a hill or go faster, and if it is too difficult, simply slow down; you can literally auto-regulate what you are doing in real time.

## Respect

While the goal of exercise is not solely to feel badass or strike fear in the hearts of men and desire in the hearts of women, you may have had enough of the church softball league or corporate kickball games. While these activities might be fun, you probably were inebriated, and they didn't make you harder to kill, help you become more functionally fit, or improve the look of your naked body. Rucking, though, will do all of that! Training like an ancient Greek hoplite warrior will increase your self-respect, and the acquisition of well-earned admiration is more satisfying than any drunk softball game.

## Helps Novices in the Gym

Besides being the holy grail of work capacity, rucking teaches you to move efficiently while under a load (talk about functional!). Moving under load is foundational to doing big things in the gym, and once you do this well, other things in the gym become easier.

## Balance and Body Awareness

Applying additional load to your shoulder blades helps improve your coordination and stability because it will make you feel more grounded. Your brain and the supporting rucking musculature become aware of the added load and must synchronize to accommodate it. This helps in sport and life.

**Final Thoughts**

Rucking allows you to combine aerobic training and strength training. As you regularly ruck, you will notice its impact on the rest of your health. Your posture improves, your stamina increases, your back pain disappears, and you look better naked!

Let's make some rucking gains!

# Chapter II

## Tactical Athletes and Load Carriage

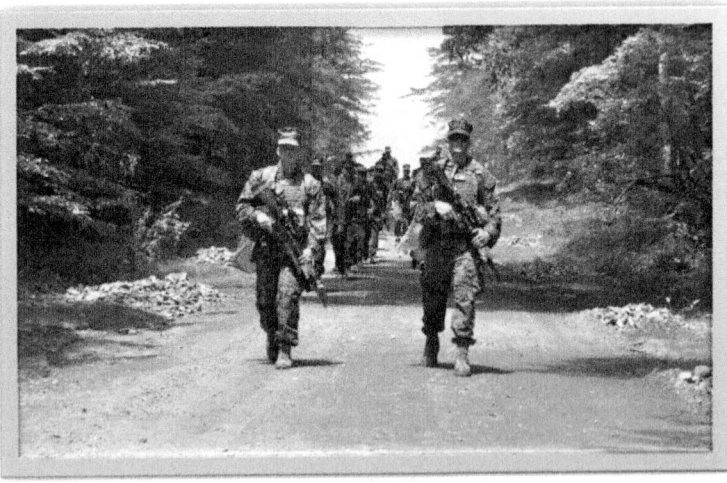

**Figure 3. Lieutenants Walker and DeRose performing a weighted hike during a Marine Officer Course.**

A half century ago, a computer was the size of a house.

Today, your smartphone is millions of times more powerful than NASA's computing abilities in 1969 (the year a man first went to the moon).

Despite the fact technology has condensed the size of "things," the required loads carried by members of the armed forces haven't fallen in line with this trend. For example, from ancient Greek warfare all the way up to the American Civil War, the overall weight carried by a warfighter was approximately 40 pounds. This means that over approximately 2,000 years, there was no significant change in the load a soldier was expected to carry.

Surprisingly, at the start of the 20th century and by World War II, the load carried by soldiers increased, drastically. Many soldiers routinely carried loads of 80 to 100 pounds. Then, for the most part, loads carried by warfighters from World War II through the Vietnam War flatlined. However, since then, they have increased faster than a sailor on a two-hour leave.

In the US operation in Grenada in 1983, some soldiers carried loads of 120 pounds or more. In the research paper *Load Carriage in Military Operations* by Joseph Knapik, ScD, and Katy Reynolds, MD, one soldier in Grenada was quoted as saying, "My rucksack weighed 120 pounds. I would get up and rush for 10 yards, throw myself down and couldn't get up. I'd rest for 10 or 15 minutes, struggle to get up, go 10 more yards, and collapse. After a few rushes, I was physically unable to move and I am in great shape."

In recent conflicts during operations in Afghanistan's rugged, mountainous terrain, some soldiers had to carry up to 140 pounds of additional external load. On average, US soldiers in the Afghanistan conflict carried 99 pounds. On the domestic front, SWAT team members routinely carry loads greater than

65 pounds, and a vast majority of cops wear more than 20 pounds of gear.

Load carriage is a universal feature of the job for tactical athletes, such as law enforcement officers, military, firefighters, and bouncers at the roughest kick 'n stab bars (we always revere the time-honored profession of the doorman).

Load carriage increases biomechanical demands on tactical athletes. In particular, there is stress placed on the back, core, lower body, and shoulders. The tension extends beyond the physical toil and into the realm of cognitive capacity. As a result of carrying a heavy load, there can be lapses in logic, situational awareness, decision-making, and mental abilities.

To develop an understanding of the weight carried by warfighters, take a look at the average loads carried by US soldiers in 2003 during dismounted operations in Afghanistan.

For reference with this table:

The fight load requires a soldier to carry all of his or her needs to defeat the enemy. While this load is heavy, the soldier still needs speed and agility to complete their mission successfully.

The approach march load is where direct contact with the enemy is in motion. The objective here is to let the soldiers fight and sustain until they are resupplied.

Emergency approach loads contain heavy items that cannot be transported by vehicle due to issues with impassable terrain.

| Duty Position | Fight Load in Pounds | Approach March Load in Pounds | Emergency Approach March Load in Pounds |
|---|---|---|---|
| Rifleman | 64 | 95 | 128 |
| Antitank Specialist | 68 | 99 | 130 |
| Weapons Squad Leader | 62 | 99 | 132 |
| Assistance Gunner | 68 | 121 | 148 |
| Ammunition Bearer | 68 | 117 | 143 |
| Platoon Medic | 55 | 92 | 119 |
| Mortar Squad Leader | 62 | 128 | 143 |
| Sapper Engineer | 60 | 95 | 132 |
| Fire Support Officer | 55 | 93 | No Data |
| Company First Sergeant | 64 | 90 | 125 |
| Rifle Company Commander | 66 | 97 | 110 |

# Training for Load Carriage

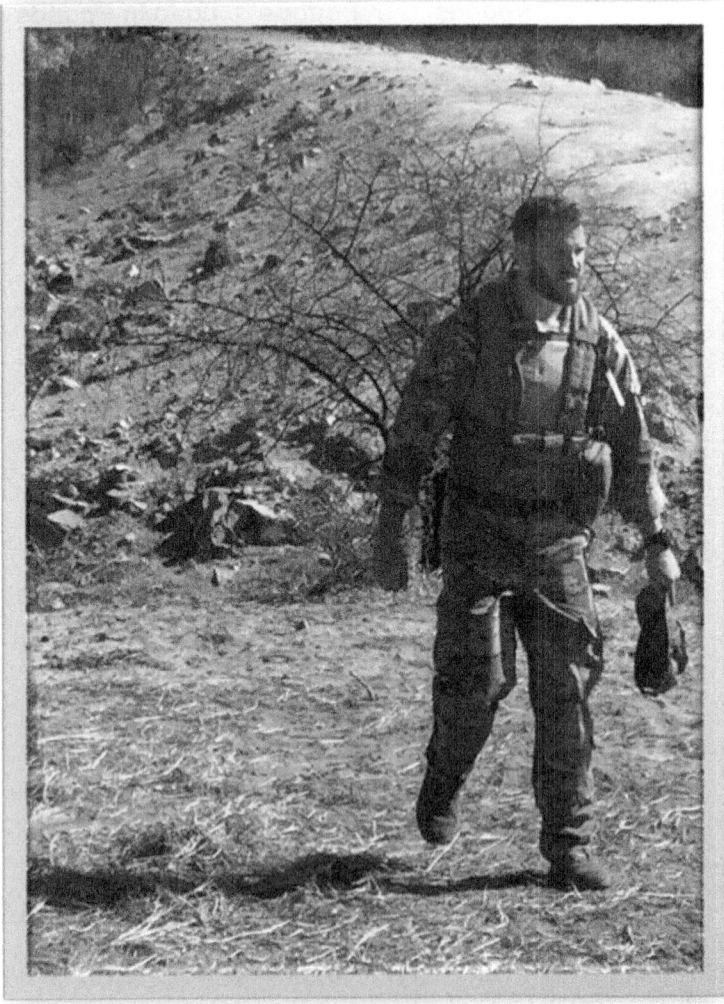

**Figure 4. Harry Walker rucking to an overwatch position while anti-poaching in South Africa.**

Due to the weight carried into a hazardous zone, experts in recent decades have focused their attention on developing programs to help tactical athletes perform optimally under load.

For example, soldiers might need to march across rugged terrain with their supplies and equipment, while being ready to move with explosivity and great agility at the drop of a hat. Sprinting (under heavy load), casualty evacuation, and many other soldiering tasks are executed quickly and under extreme load.

The success of military and law enforcement operations often depends on the speed, mobility, and conditioning levels they can display under load.

SO, PLEASE NOTE:

If you are specifically training for your job and the stakes are life or death, it is recommended that you train and exercise with load distributions and load totality similar to your vocation. This is the principle of specificity in action.

The Army defines readiness as the capability of its forces to conduct the full range of military operations, including the defeat of all enemies, regardless of the threats they pose. This readiness, in large part, is dependent on the physical readiness of the tactical athletes within a unit.

Okay, what about you?

For you, readiness might mean spotting and stalking a black bear in the Sierra Blanca mountains while adhering to fair chase rules and then successfully transporting your kill back to base camp. Or, it could mean successfully removing some passed-out roughnecks who rented out the local Elks lodge for a birthday party. Or, maybe, you have to transport a 40-pound sleeping toddler without a stroller.

Readiness is having the ability to meet and thrive in whatever situation you encounter. It's what we call being Gas Station Ready.

The bottom line: If you follow what's laid out in rucking gains and prepare yourself to move for prolonged periods of time under load, you will be ready!

## Training for Rucking

Since the 1990s, there has been an effort to develop programming strategies for tactical athletes to condition for load carriage. A review of the literature proposes that most effective modalities for improving load carriage performance are a combination of aerobic, strength training, and load-carriage-specific exercises.

At any time, tactical athletes must be ready to march across rugged terrain with their supplies and equipment. From an operational planning standpoint, it is imperative that the military is able to predict the ability of warfighters to handle prolonged load-carriage tasks.

Traditional aerobic tasks have a large bias against heavier tactical athletes. Both body mass and body composition are important variables to examine for load carriage because high amounts of lean body mass and low percentages of body fat have been shown to improve load-carriage ability. While increases in lean mass increase load-carriage ability, increases in body fat impair it. Strength, muscle hypertrophy, optimal body composition, and a strong aerobic base will help the tactical athlete excel in load-carriage tasks. The limiting factors for performing well with load carriage are strength and power production capabilities; in other words, the marathon runner with a Peewee Herman–like physique is not built to thrive in load-carriage tasks.

In reality, tactical athletes need muscle hypertrophy, not just to strike fear in the hearts of potential assailants, but also because strength, low body fat, and a strong aerobic base will help them perform well under load.

In fact, the purpose of the rucking gains program is to get stronger, become leaner, perform better, and look better.

Rucking will get you looking Chippendales Ready, while staying Gas Station Ready.

# Chapter III

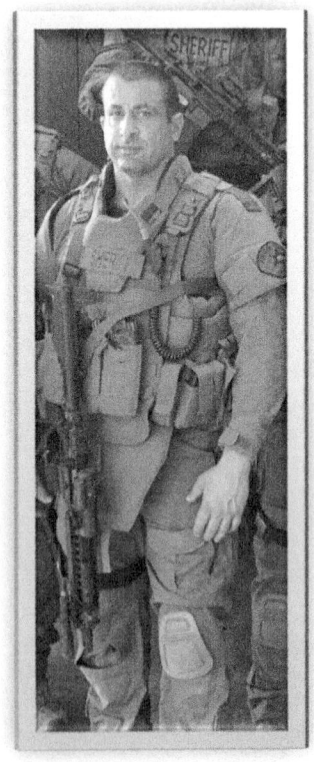

**Figure 5. Taylor Lopes trains to be able to move well in SWAT gear.**

Following "Lombardi time" (if you're not early, you're late), we sat on a bench overlooking the beachscape and waited for Deano.

In preparation for our first ruck with Deano, we followed his specific instructions. First, we headed to our local Supply Sergeant army surplus store and bought some old military issue rucksacks. We loaded sand into plastic bags and piled them into those old, durable backpacks. Then, using the scale at the gym, we made sure that the packs were 10 percent of our bodyweight.

As far as footwear went, we made sure our well-worn and comfortable athletic shoes (neither of us had boots) were carefully and tightly tied. Our socks were new and made from a synthetic material.

When Deano came over to our bench, we were actively engaged in that most important activity for the situationally aware: people watching.

An alert vet of foreign wars in faraway lands, Deano knew the importance of tracking, watching, and monitoring the human animal. He gave a tacit nod in acknowledgment and approval for how we were spending our time.

"Watching people, learning their traits, and observing subtle actions is time well spent," Deano said as a greeting.

"What do you see?" he asked.

"People walking."

"Beyond that. What do you see?"

"People, they walk differently."

"Go on," Deano said, coaxing us to continue.

"Well, that lady, the one over there," we said, pointing to a Hollywood type in an oversized floppy beach hat, "she is, um, hesitant, or cautious, before every step."

"What does that tell you?"

"She is hesitant, uncertain about her next step, her decisions."

"Good, good. What else do you see?"

"That one guy, the one in the baseball hat and oversized trunks."

"Yeah, what about him?"

"His shoulders, they're slouched. His posture, it's not very good. You can really tell that the guy doesn't have a lot of confidence, that he doesn't believe in himself."

"Good eye. Anyone else?"

"Sure, that guy way down there with the pumped-up arms but no legs."

Deano gave a very slight chuckle, but said nothing. So we continued.

"His walk, he, um, takes steps that stretch beyond the natural movement of his body. The steps are so long that he keeps hitting the ground with his heel. The guy thinks his capacity is greater than it is. He has an ego, maybe even some degree of narcissism."

"Yeah, so what does this teach you?"

"How you walk, it matters."

"It sure does. Now, I'm going to take you boys on a ruck. And it's going to really matter how you move, because we will be moving with intention.

"Don't hesitate with any of your steps. Find your stride and from there let the movement happen. Pretty soon, you will find there is a meditative quality to rucking. Repetitive action performed with intention can be mind clearing and opening."

He stopped for a moment to see if the mystical talk caused us to chuckle or lose focus. It didn't. So he continued.

"Keep your shoulders back, your chest open, and your posture strong. This will improve breathing capacity, harden your core, and prevent possible injuries.

"Along the lines of preventing injury, pay attention to the length of your stride and how your foot hits the ground. Don't let your legs get too far in front of you. Use your glutes to control each step. When your foot hits the ground, do it with your midsole, not your heel. Doing this can prevent undue strain on your knees. That's going to matter more as you age.

"Okay, last thing. Keep up. We're moving at a pace of a 15-minute mile."

With that, Deano took us from the beach to the hillside of the front country, and we found the seemingly miraculous physical and spiritual benefits of the simple act of the ruck.

## Rucking Guidelines

This a journey where you will be moving with intention, keeping a brisk pace with an external load for the specific purpose of physical training. To keep you safe and to maximize results, we have put together rucking guidelines.

If you want to take your rucking to the next level, we recommend you follow the periodized programs we have provided.

Want to improve your aesthetics, health, and aerobic conditioning as well as build your work capacity? Then simply follow the guidelines presented. Alongside your existing strength training routine, this will work like a charm!

## Boots and Foot Care

The success of a military mission frequently depends on the ability of troops to access a remote area on foot. And as we covered, the external loads carried by soldiers have increased over time.

In recent deployments, soldiers, because of the increased load carriage demands they face while wearing boots, have experienced increased repetitive stress on their bones, muscles, and nerves, which has increased the likelihood of injuries. The lower extremities (knees, lower legs, ankles, and feet) and back are the most affected; some of the specific injuries include:

- Foot blisters
- Knee injuries
- Ankle injuries
- Back strains and injuries
- Stress fractures
- Nerve compression injuries

For occupational or training purposes, we offer the following tips for wearing boots:

## Foot care tips while on military missions or training in boots

- Make sure your boots are properly fitted.
- Wear synthetic socks that are not too tight or too loose (cotton ones shrink and don't manage moisture well).
- Layer your socks by wearing a slippery pair of socks under a heavier pair of socks to decrease friction.
- Buy new socks when you get new boots.
- Let your boots "air out" when your feet are not in them.
- Take your time breaking in a new pair of boots.
- Apply adhesive products such as moleskin (adhesive flannel), athletic tape, pressure pads, or blister bandages over sensitive areas, such as your toes and heels, before putting on your socks.
- Practice good foot hygiene.
- Keep your feet as dry as possible.
- Keep your toenails cut short and straight.

- Inspect your feet regularly for blisters, sores, or any potential injury.
- Rest your feet after being in boots for hours.

You can avoid virtually all rucking-related injuries with the guidelines presented in this chapter.

## Rucking Footwear Options

What are the best shoes for rucking? There is a lot of back and forth online about this topic, but when making your decision, be sure to sniff out the potential agenda like shit on a shoe.

Usually, someone online is trying to sell you something or get you to join Uncle Fester's latest Ponzi Scheme; remember, there is a reason Fester is more broke than the Ten Commandments.

While boots are commonly used for rucking, the truth is the best rucking shoes are the ones that feel the best to you. Some people prefer running shoes like Brooks or Salomon, others tactical boots. Any athletic shoe that is comfortable on your feet is going to work well for rucking. Don't break the bank rucking; use what's already in your closet before buying something new.

Boots are most helpful when you are going really heavy or for really long, 20+ mile rucks. Boots are also useful for uneven terrain because of the added ankle stability. In those situations, you really want your heel locked in place to avoid hot spots and blisters.

While you have some leeway in choosing footwear, there are some options that should be off the table. Don't ruck in Birkenstocks, aka Jesus Sandals, or cowboy boots; find a comfortable athletic shoe and get going.

## Rucksack/Backpack/Weighted Vest

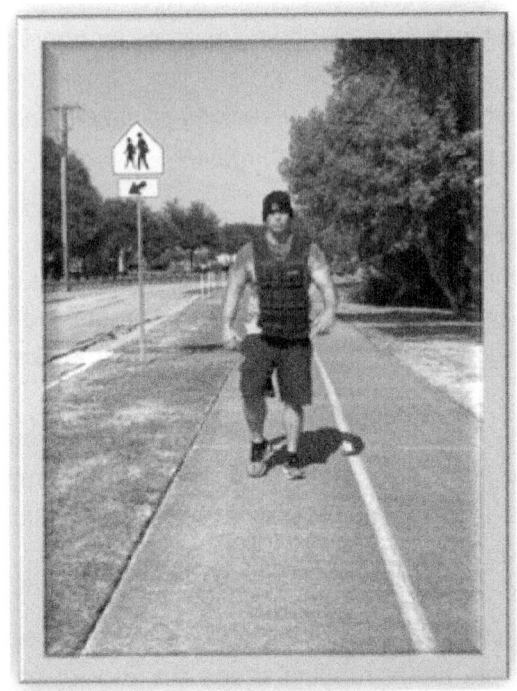

**Figure 6. Josh Bryant is not only the president but also a client.**

You can absolutely just throw some weights in a well-fitted backpack and start making some rucking gains. If you're doing this for occupational demands or to pass a specific assessment, remember the principle of specificity discussed earlier.

A good rucksack/backpack for rucking fits your torso; the top should rest on your shoulders, and the bottom should end before the top of your butt. This ensures your stride will not be obstructed as you walk. The backpack should have a rigid frame to support the ruck's weight and distribute the load across your back.

The backpack needs to have shoulder straps, seams, and padding that are built to hold heavy loads comfortably. The backpack's cloth should be durable and made to handle heavy loads, such as 1000D Cordura. Stress points in the shoulder straps, handles, and seams should be sewn with high-tensile thread. Military rucksacks at army surplus stores work great and will save you cash. Wide, well-padded straps will help the ruck feel much more comfortable.

Some rucksacks and backpacks have a padded waist belt that transfers the load to your hips; cinching this strap is the most secure way to carry. Adjust your shoulder straps and sternum strap to anchor the load to the small of your back, which will reduce swinging. You want to keep the weight close and stable.

Of course, for fitness purposes, a well-fitted weight vest will get the job done.

## Physical Preparedness

In the military, it has been found that low fitness levels correspond with an increase in the risk of injury during general training and that this risk is intensified during load-carriage tasks. What does this mean to someone training for combat or the civilian looking to improve her aesthetics for the upcoming apartment complex toga and pool party?

Plain and simple, you gotta get in shape to ruck.

Do not go from zero to hero—you must be in shape to ruck. As military research consistently shows, physical training to increase fitness levels decreases load-carriage injuries.

Preparing soldiers to carry loads goes way back to the Roman legionnaires. Alas, even with these thousands of years of experience, practical guidelines on how to prepare for rucking are virtually nonexistent.

Research shows that other supplementary strength and conditioning modalities, such as lifting weights, are beneficial. Increases in rucking weight, rucking speed, the percentage of a grade on a hill, and even the difficulty of terrain you are rucking will increase energy expenditure and should be used as an intensity metric.

For example, an increase in speed of 0.5 km/h (or 0.31 MPH) or an increase in incline grade of just 1 percent have both been revealed to have a comparable energy expenditure effect as carrying an additional 10 kilograms of load (22 pounds).

Here is the bottom line: Increasing the speed of a ruck or the angle of incline has a very similar physiological effect to increasing ruck weight, hence increasing the intensity level.

Remember this: Rome was not built in a day.

Keep in mind the progressive overload principle, which says that over time, continually increasing the demands on your musculoskeletal system will allow you to continually make gains in muscle size, strength, and endurance. Over time, the intensity of rucking should be gradually increased for the civilian to meet his goal and for the tactical athlete to meet her occupational demands.

## Rucking Warm-Up

Admittedly, many folks just throw on a pack or vest and immediately begin rucking. However, to optimize the process and reduce the risk of injury, we recommend a five-minute general warm-up, which should be any activity that elevates the heart rate for five minutes: walking fast, jogging, cardio machine, whatever.

Next, follow either one of the Jailhouse Strong dynamic warm-ups on YouTube.

Now, walk at a mild pace for three to five minutes with the load you will be rucking with.

Now it's time to ruck!

## Rucking Technique

Before you head out on your first ruck, read through the following technique guidelines to stay safe and get the most out of your workout.

First, you need to be able to walk regularly before you can start rucking, and you should never run while rucking, which would put astronomical amounts of stress on your joints and could lead to injury. That being said, rucking with great technique as outlined here will save your back, knees, and hips while simultaneously building core strength and reinforcing good posture!

Keep in mind that there's no need to exceed a 15-minute mile ruck pace unless you're training for a specialized assessment (we will reiterate this point throughout this book).

Follow these tips while rucking:

- Keep your head high and spine aligned and stand tall. If you cannot maintain optimal posture, you are going too heavy.
- Anti-shrug your shoulders and continually check to see if you are rounding your shoulders or shrugging them up. Keep your shoulders down and back, but don't do it to the extent you are pulling hard. If you must round or shrug, you are going too heavy.
- Avoid overextension or spinal flexion; maintain a neutral midline.
- Stay upright, achieving full extension of your hips while walking.

- Shorten your strides to keep the close foot striking closer to underneath your hip; use more frequent strides while driving your arms hard.
- Walk with your butt, and no buts about it! Keep your glutes engaged; this is done by flexing your glutes to power through the movement.
- Step with flat feet, shooting for a midfoot instead of a heel strike. This will save your knees.
- Avoid pounding your feet by trying a "glide stride"; this keeps a smooth momentum moving forward and saves your knees, so one foot is always touching the ground.

While this is not as complex as mastering the snatch, we are talking Olympic lifting, lothario. Proper technique will ensure the benefits of rucking and eliminate most of the risk.

## Rucking Terrain

It's better to just ruck around your suburban subdivision than not ruck. However, we recommend getting out in nature or going to the beach, if possible, to fully reap the mental health benefits.

According to the American Psychiatric Association, 39 percent of adults are more anxious than they were a year ago and suicide rates have greatly increased during the COVID pandemic. We are not mental health professionals but do recommend doing what provides the greatest mental health boosts, as long as you don't sacrifice training quality.

For general fitness, just get out and enjoy nature. It's a challenge to navigate the natural terrain. Guided trails are everywhere; there are apps you can use, or you can create your own trail. Just avoid busy roads.

If you are training for a job-specific test, do your best to find terrain similar to where the test will be administered.

## Rucking Weight/Distance/Frequency

Assuming you don't go apeshit, rucking can help improve your recovery because it builds an aerobic base, which is essential for regeneration and serves as an active recovery. For example, the day after a heavy deadlift workout, a moderate ruck could absolutely serve as an active recovery session.

Assuming the goal is improving health and conditioning, start with 20 to 30 minutes of rucking. Assuming you have a decent baseline of conditioning (which you need to), shoot for 20-minute miles on a flat surface or very low incline. Start with 5 to 10 percent of your bodyweight. For general fitness, you do not need to exceed 10 percent of your bodyweight, but for someone with a great level of conditioning and capable of a double bodyweight squat or deadlift and a sub 15 percent body fat percentage, it is okay to go up to as much as 20 percent of your bodyweight. Do not exceed this.

You can increase one of the following variables each week:

- Increase ruck weight up to five pounds (never exceeding 20 percent of bodyweight)
- Increase distance rucked a quarter mile
- Increase five minutes in total duration in a week
- Increase incline grade 2 percent
- Ruck on a more difficult surface, such as soft sand versus a synthetic track

For pure general health purposes, nasal breathing is an excellent guideline; you'll want to maintain a pace you can keep without breathing out of your mouth or one where you are working but are still able to keep a conversation going. Simply keeping your heart rate between 110 to 145 beats per minute for the ruck will also do the trick.

To reap most of the benefits and essentially make rucking almost risk-free, we recommend a total of 60 minutes a week with 10 percent of your bodyweight or less. These 60 minutes can be divided into one or two sessions, all while rucking at a pace you can carry on a conversation at. You never have to progress pass this point, unless you are looking for performance or tactical job simulation training.

## The Eight Commandments of Rucking

Make sure you do not break rucking's eight commandments:

I.  **Walk before you ruck.** You should not be rucking if you are not regularly walking or running. Minimally, walk every day for 30 minutes. You should be able to easily walk for 60 minutes straight at a brisk pace.

II. **Use progressive overload.** No matter how high your fitness level is, progress slowly by adding no more than five pounds a week to your ruck or weighted vest.

III. **Do not run while rucking.** Maintain a brisk, intentional walk; the benefit of running under the stress of a load does not come close to justifying the risk.

IV. **If you do not train your lower body with weights, you do not need to be rucking.** You need minimally six months of foundational training with barbell core movements before rucking. (The Jailhouse Strong Pig Iron Program is a great place to start.)

V.  **Do not ruck daily.** Your rucks should be limited to two a week maximum; for military training purposes, two to four times a month spread evenly have been shown to have immense benefits.

VI.  **Take care of your feet.**

VII.  **Do not exceed a 15-minute mile pace.**

VIII. **Be patient and trust the process.** Follow these guidelines so you are properly prepared for rucking.

## Final Thoughts

Rucking has grown in popularity but has failed to go totally mainstream because rucking doesn't make an equipment manufacturer rich, cause a chain gym to gain thousands of sign-ups, or line the pockets of some pseudo-famous personal trainer.

Rucking benefits you and only you.

Following the guidelines presented, you can add rucking to your existing fitness or strength programs; it will make you healthy, harder to kill, and stronger.

Let's make some rucking gains.

# Chapter IV

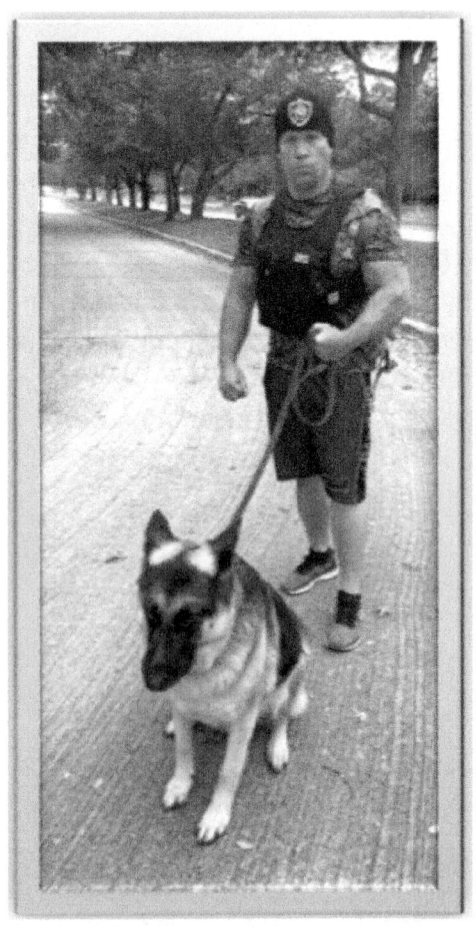

**Figure 7. Josh Bryant, accompanied by Duke, on a ruck.**

## The Rucking Gains Program

In the preceding chapters, you have learned about rucking and its benefits as well as the guidelines that go into program design. From here, you can absolutely design your own rucking program, and we have included a review of the Seven Granddaddy Laws of Training to guide your potential program design and let you see what goes into our design.

## The Seven Granddaddy Laws of Training

The Seven Granddaddy Laws of training were categorized by the late Dr. Fred Hatfield. These are the guiding principles in program design.

1. **The Law of Individual Differences:** We all have different bodies, abilities, and weaknesses, and we all respond differently (to a degree) to any given system of training. These differences should be taken into consideration when designing your training program. Try the programs we have laid out and, over time, customize them to yourself.

2. **The Overcompensation Principle:** Mother Nature overcompensates for training stress by increasing fitness levels, assuming adequate recovery.

3. **The Overload Principle:** To make Mother Nature overcompensate, you must stress your muscles beyond what they're already used to. Notice the progression in our included programs.

4. **The SAID Principle:** The acronym stands for Specific Adaptation to Imposed Demands. Each organ and organelle responds to a different form of stress.

5. **The Use/Disuse Principle:** "Use it or lose it"; to keep your rucking gains, you must keep on rucking, just like

the bodybuilder must keep on lifting for hypertrophy to keep muscularity.

6. **The GAS Principle:** The acronym for General Adaptation Syndrome, this law states that there must be a period of low-intensity training or complete rest following periods of high-intensity training. Take a look at the "reload weeks" in the rucking programs included in this book.

7. **The Specificity Principle:** You'll get more efficient at rucking by rucking as opposed to swimming, for example.

## The Program

We have included a 16-week training protocol designed specifically to improve your rucking. The program is designed to be executed once a week; admittedly, people have done it twice a week without issue. However, once a week is the safe bet.

You can run this program in conjunction with an existing strength program or follow the strength training program included later in this book, in conjunction with the 16-week rucking gains program, to produce synergistic results.

| Week | Training Protocol | Notes |
|------|-------------------|-------|
| 1 | Ruck for 20 minutes with 6% of bodyweight. | Stay on flat ground, ruck at a 20-minute mile pace. |
| 2 | Ruck for 25 minutes with 8% of bodyweight. | Stay on flat ground, ruck at a 19-minute mile pace. |
| 3 | Ruck for 25 minutes with 10% of bodyweight. | Stay on flat ground, ruck at an 18-minute mile pace. |
| 4 | Ruck for 30 minutes with 12% of bodyweight. | Stay on flat ground, ruck at a 17-minute mile pace. |
| 5 | Ruck for 33 minutes with 14% of bodyweight. | Stay on flat ground, ruck at a 16-minute mile pace. |

| 6 | Ruck for 36 minutes with 16% of bodyweight. | Stay on flat ground, ruck at a 15-minute mile pace. |
|---|---|---|
| 7 | Ruck for 40 minutes with 18% of bodyweight. | Stay on flat ground, ruck at a 15-minute mile pace. |
| 8 | Ruck for 30 minutes with 15% of bodyweight. | Stay on flat ground, ruck at a 15-minute mile pace. This is a reload week. |
| 9 | Ruck for 45 minutes with 18% of bodyweight. | Stay on flat ground, ruck at a 15-minute mile pace. |
| 10 | Ruck for 45 minutes with 20% of bodyweight. | Stay on flat ground, ruck at a 15-minute mile pace. |
| 11 | Ruck for 45 minutes with 20% of bodyweight. | Introduce low rolling hills, ruck at a 15-minute mile pace. |
| 12 | Ruck for 50 minutes with 20% of bodyweight. | Increase steepness of hills, ruck at a 15-minute mile pace. |
| 13 | Ruck for 55 minutes with 20% of bodyweight. | Same hills as last week, ruck at a 15-minute mile pace. |
| 14 | Ruck for 60 minutes with 20% of bodyweight. | Same hills as last week, ruck at a 15-minute mile pace. |
| 15 | Ruck for 60 minutes with 20% of bodyweight. | Increase steepness of hills, ruck at a 15-minute mile pace. |
| 16 | Ruck for 30 minutes with 20% of bodyweight. | Stay on flat ground, ruck at a 15-minute mile pace. This is a reload week. |

## Strength Program

The program is laid out in four-week cycles, as shown below. For bench press supplementary exercises, squat supplementary movements, chest exercises, arm exercises, rowing exercises, and hamstring exercises, pick from the list below, but remember to follow the specified-rep protocols. These movements should be performed with maximum intensity and rotated every one to four weeks. You are given freedom to make the program fit your individual specifications. However, stick to the core movements. If it is easy to lift the weight, do it more explosively or do more reps on sets where you are prescribed to hit a maximum number of reps. But never go heavy on the reload because this is when active recovery allows for the largest strength and muscle gains to take place.

After a four-week cycle is completed (three weeks of buildup training and the one-week reload), start over. At the beginning of each four-week cycle, add five pounds to each core lift; or if you feel ambitious, add 10 pounds. Never more! Do this as long as possible. You can retest your maxes after three four-week cycles. Of course, max out after the reload week so that your body is fresh and rested! If these jumps seem small, then lift the weight more explosively and do more reps. You will get stronger.

**Frequency**

On paper, this program appears to be three days a week. Always rest at least 48 hours between days one and two, as well as between days two and three, and then again between days three and one. Remember, a week is a man-made concept; it has nothing to do with physiology or how you adapt to training. If you recover slowly, make your week eight or nine days; if you recover quickly, do five or six days. The majority of people will hit the sweet spot with a seven-day week.

# Exercise Choices

## Bench Press Supplementary

Board Presses (1-5)

Loaded Push-Up Variations

Weighted Dips

Floor Press

Dead Bench Press (Dead Bench is single repetitions only; for supplementary work, 3 to 8 singles are appropriate.)

Close-Grip Incline Press

## Squat Supplementary

Front Squats

Pause Squats

Olympic Pause Squats

Zercher Squats

Overhead Squats

Dead Squats (Dead Squats are single repetitions only; for supplementary work, 3 to 8 singles are appropriate.)

Step-Ups

Belt Squats

Lunges

## Chest

Incline Dumbbell/Cable Fly

Flat Dumbbell/Cable Fly

Decline Dumbbell/Cable Fly

Band Fly

Dumbbell/Barbell Pull Over

Hammer-Grip Dumbbell Bench Press

Any Chest Machine

## Biceps

Zottman Curls
Barbell 21 Curls
Dumbbell Incline Curls (big stretch, palms supinated whole time)
Reverse Curls
EZ-Curl Bar Curls
Hammer Curls
Towel Kettlebell Curls
Spider Curls
Any Biceps Machine

## Triceps

Barbell Floor Paused Triceps Extensions
Skull Crushers
Rolling Dumbbell Triceps Extensions
French Press
JM Press
Dick's Press
Triceps Pushdowns
Band Triceps Pushdowns
Any Triceps Machine

## Rowing Variations

Dead-Stop Bent-Over Rows
Reverse-Grip Rows
One-Armed Dumbbell Rows
Head-Supported Rows
T-Bar Prison Rows
Meadows Rows
Seal Rows

Seated Rows
Any Horizontal Pulling Machine

## Hamstrings
Leg Curls
One-Leg Deadlifts
Romanian Deadlifts
Glute Ham Raises
Pull Throughs
Nordic Leg Curls
Inverse Leg Curls
Band Leg Curls

## Week 1

## Day 1

| Exercise | Weight | Sets | Reps | Special Notes |
|---|---|---|---|---|
| Squats | 70% | 3 | 10,8, Max | Last set, do as many reps as possible, but do not go to failure, finish one rep shy. |
| Squat Supplementary Lift | | 2 | 5-8 | |
| Hamstring Exercise | | 4-5 | 5-8 | |
| Max body-weight squats 90 seconds | Bodyweight | 1 | Max | Strive to improve reps rather than time. |

Continue

| Exercise | Weight | Sets | Reps | Special Notes |
|---|---|---|---|---|
| Standing Weighted Crunches | | 5 | 10-15 | |
| Neck Extensions | | 2 | 20 | |

## Day 2

| Exercise | Weight | Sets | Reps | Special Notes |
|---|---|---|---|---|
| Bench Press | 70% | 3 | 10,8,Max | Last set rest-pause 20. The number specifies the rest interval between sets of rest-pause. Do as many reps as possible, rest 20 seconds. Repeat, resting 20 seconds between each set of rest-pause. Do not go to failure, finish one rep shy. |
| Bench Press Supplementary Lift | | 2-3 | 6-10 | |
| Chest Exercise | | 3 | 10-15 | |
| Triceps Exercise | | 4 | 10-15 | |

| | | | | |
|---|---|---|---|---|
| **Pull-up or chin-up variation** | | 3 | 5-10 | Add weight if you can do more than 10 reps. If you cannot do pull-ups, do band-assisted or lat pulldowns (or any other vertical pulling motion). |
| **Neck Flexions** | | 2 | 20 | |

## Day 3

| Exercise | Weight | Sets | Reps | Special Notes |
|---|---|---|---|---|
| **Deadlifts** | 90% | 1 | 2 | |
| **Speed Deadlifts** | 75% | 6 | 3 | Rest 90-120 seconds between sets |
| **Overhead Press** | 80% | 1 | RP | Rest-pause 20. The number specifies the rest interval between sets of rest-pause. Do as many reps as possible, rest 20 seconds. Repeat, resting 20 seconds between each set of rest-pause. Do not go to failure, finish one rep shy. |
| **Snatch Grip Shrugs** | | 3 | 10-20 | |

Continue

| Exercise | Weight | Sets | Reps | Special Notes |
|---|---|---|---|---|
| **Total Rep Method Chin-ups 100** | | ?? | ?? | Go to failure on each set. Once you can do this in 12 sets, add 10 lbs. Each time this is achieved, add 10 more pounds. |
| **Row Exercise** | | 3 | 5-8 | Barbell or dumbbells |
| **Biceps Exercise** | | 4 | 10-15 | |
| **Side Necks** | | 2 | 20 | |

## Week 2

## Day 1

| Exercise | Weight | Sets | Reps | Special Notes |
|---|---|---|---|---|
| **Squats** | 80% | 3 | 5,5, Max | Last set, do as many reps as possible, but do not go to failure, finish one rep shy. |
| **Squat Supplementary Lift** | | 2 | 5-8 | |
| **Hamstring Exercise** | | 4-5 | 5-8 | |
| **Max body-weight squats 90 seconds** | Bodyweight | 1 | Max | Strive to improve reps rather than time. |

| Exercise | | Sets | Reps | |
|---|---|---|---|---|
| Standing Weighted Crunches | | 5 | 10-15 | |
| Neck Extensions | | 2 | 20 | |

## Day 2

| Exercise | Weight | Sets | Reps | Special Notes |
|---|---|---|---|---|
| Bench Press | 80% | 3 | 5,5,Max | Last set rest-pause 20. The number specifies the rest interval between sets of rest-pause. Do as many reps as possible, rest 20 seconds. Repeat, resting 20 seconds between each set of rest-pause. Do not go to failure, finish one rep shy. |
| Bench Press Supplementary Lift | | 2-3 | 6-10 | |
| Chest Exercise | | 3 | 10-15 | |
| Triceps Exercise | | 4 | 10-15 | |

Continue

| Exercise | Weight | Sets | Reps | Special Notes |
|---|---|---|---|---|
| **Pull-up or chin-up variation** | | 3 | 5-10 | Add weight if you can do more than 10 reps. If you cannot do pull-ups, do band-assisted or lat pulldowns (or any other vertical pulling motion). |
| **Neck Flexions** | | 2 | 20 | |

## Day 3

| Exercise | Weight | Sets | Reps | Special Notes |
|---|---|---|---|---|
| **Deadlifts** | 75% | 15 | 1 | Rest 30 seconds between sets. |
| **Overhead Press** | 82.5% | 1 | RP | Rest-pause 20. The number specifies the rest interval between sets of rest-pause. Do as many reps as possible, rest 20 seconds. Repeat, resting 20 seconds between each set of rest-pause. Do not go to failure, finish one rep shy. |
| **Snatch Grip Shrugs** | | 3 | 10-20 | |

| | | | | |
|---|---|---|---|---|
| **Total Rep Method Chin-ups 100** | | ?? | ?? | Go to failure on each set. Once you can do this in 12 sets, add 10 lbs. Each time this is achieved, add 10 more pounds. |
| **Row Exercise** | | 3 | 5-8 | Barbell or dumbbells |
| **Biceps Exercise** | | 4 | 10-15 | |
| **Side Necks** | | 2 | 20 | |

## Week 3

## Day 1

| Exercise | Weight | Sets | Reps | Special Notes |
|---|---|---|---|---|
| **Squats** | 85% | 3 | 3,3, Max | Last set, do as many reps as possible, but do not go to failure, finish one rep shy. |
| **Squat Supplementary Lift** | | 2 | 5-8 | |
| **Hamstring Exercise** | | 4-5 | 5-8 | |
| **Max body-weight squats 90 seconds** | Bodyweight | 1 | Max | Strive to improve reps rather than time. |

Continue

| Exercise | Weight | Sets | Reps | Special Notes |
|---|---|---|---|---|
| Standing Weighted Crunches | | 5 | 10-15 | |
| Neck Extensions | | 2 | 20 | |

## Day 2

| Exercise | Weight | Sets | Reps | Special Notes |
|---|---|---|---|---|
| Bench Press | 85% | 3 | 3,3,Max | Last set rest-pause 20. The number specifies the rest interval between sets of rest-pause. Do as many reps as possible, rest 20 seconds. Repeat, resting 20 seconds between each set of rest-pause. Do not go to failure, finish one rep shy. |
| Bench Press Supplementary Lift | | 2-3 | 6-10 | |
| Chest Exercise | | 3 | 10-15 | |

| | | | | |
|---|---|---|---|---|
| **Triceps Exercise** | | 4 | 10-15 | |
| **Pull-up or chin-up variation** | | 3 | 5-10 | Add weight if you can do more than 10 reps. If you cannot do pull-ups, do band-assisted or lat pulldowns (or any other vertical pulling motion). |
| **Neck Flexions** | | 2 | 20 | |

## Day 3

| Exercise | Weight | Sets | Reps | Special Notes |
|---|---|---|---|---|
| **Deadlifts** | 80% | 6 | 2 | Rest 90-120 seconds between sets. |
| **Overhead Press** | 85% | 1 | RP | Rest-pause 20. The number specifies the rest interval between sets of rest-pause. Do as many reps as possible, rest 20 seconds. Repeat, resting 20 seconds between each set of rest-pause. Do not go to failure, finish one rep shy. |

Continue

| Exercise | Weight | Sets | Reps | Special Notes |
|---|---|---|---|---|
| Snatch Grip Shrugs | | 3 | 10-20 | |
| Total Rep Method Chin-ups 100 | | ?? | ?? | Go to failure on each set. Once you can do this in 12 sets, add 10 lbs. Each time this is achieved, add 10 more pounds. |
| Row Exercise | | 3 | 5-8 | Barbell or dumbbells |
| Biceps Exercise | | 4 | 10-15 | |
| Side Necks | | 2 | 20 | |

## Week 4 (Reload/Deload Week)

## Day 1

| Exercise | Weight | Sets | Reps | Special Notes |
|---|---|---|---|---|
| Squats | 75% | 3 | 3 | |
| Squat Supplementary Lift | | 2 | 5-8 | 70% of Week 3 Weight |
| Hamstring Exercise | | 2 | 5-8 | 70% of Week 3 Weight |
| Standing Weighted Crunches | | 3 | 10-15 | 70% of Week 3 Weight |
| Neck Extensions | | 2 | 20 | 70% of Week 3 Weight |

## Day 2

| Exercise | Weight | Sets | Reps | Special Notes |
|---|---|---|---|---|
| Bench Press | 75% | 3 | 3 | 70% of Week 3 Weight |
| Bench Press Supplementary Lift | | 2 | 6-10 | 70% of Week 3 Weight |
| Chest Exercise | | 2 | 10-15 | 70% of Week 3 Weight |
| Triceps Exercise | | 3 | 10-15 | 70% of Week 3 Weight |
| Pull-up or chin-up variation | | 3 | 5-10 | 70% of Week 3 Weight |
| Neck Flexions | | 2 | 20 | 70% of Week 3 Weight |

## Day 3

| Exercise | Weight | Sets | Reps | Special Notes |
|---|---|---|---|---|
| Deadlifts | 65% | 3 | 3 | |
| Overhead Press | 70% | 3 | 3 | 70% of Week 3 Weight |
| Snatch Grip Shrugs | | 3 | 10-20 | 70% of Week 3 Weight |
| Chin up | | 3 | 3 | Same as Week 3 Weight |
| Row Exercise | | 2 | 5-8 | 70% of Week 3 Weight |
| Biceps Exercise | | 3 | 10-15 | 70% of Week 3 Weight |
| Side Necks | | 2 | 20 | 70% of Week 3 Weight |

After the four-week routine is completed, add five pounds, or 10 pounds if you feel ambitious, to the core lift and repeat. If something is easy, do the movement more explosively or add repetitions on your max sets and rest-pauses, but do not add additional weight.

## Military Load Carriage Program

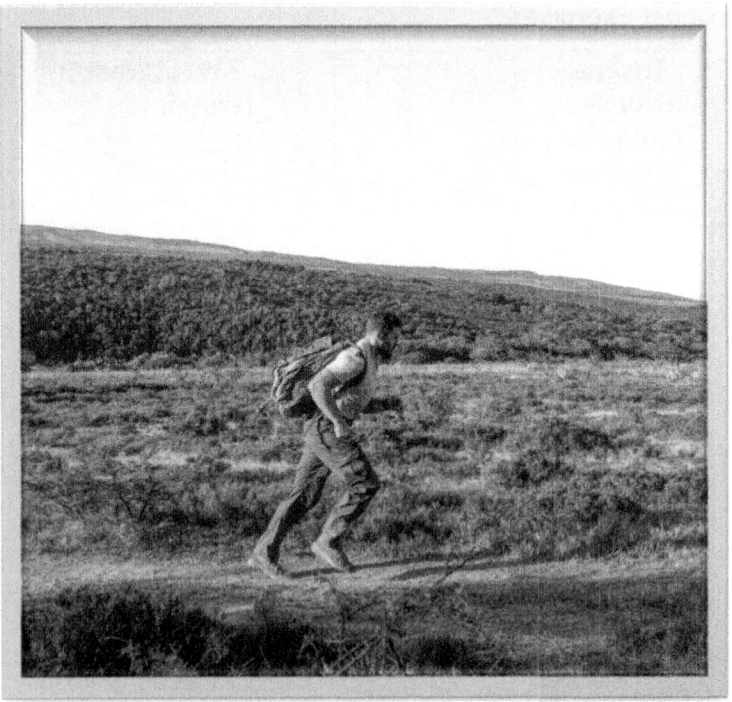

**Figure 8. Harry Walker uphill rucking.**

Below we have included an example of a 12-week program specifically designed for a soldier who will work up to doing battle simulation tasks with 65 pounds of additional load over this time frame. This would also work very well for a hunter preparing for a hunt in mountainous regions.

The training protocol below is to be executed once weekly; admittedly, some have done twice weekly without issues.

| Week | Training Protocol | Comments |
|---|---|---|
| 1 | Walk around with 25 pounds of additional load without weapon for 20 minutes at three to four miles per hour on flat ground. | |
| 2 | Walk around with 25 pounds of additional load with weapon for 20 minutes at three to four miles per hour in an area with low rolling hills. | |
| 3 | Walk around with 30 pounds of additional load with weapon for 24 minutes at three to four miles per hour in an area with low rolling hills. | Introduce weapon carriage with basic obstacles for 10 minutes. |
| 4 | Walk around with 35 pounds of additional load with weapon for 25 minutes at three to four miles per hour in an area with low rolling hills. | |
| 5 | Walk around with 40 pounds of additional load with weapon for 27 minutes at three to four miles per hour in an area with low rolling hills. | Continue weapon carriage with revised obstacles. |
| 6 | Walk around with 25 pounds of additional load with weapon for 20 minutes at three to four miles per hour in an area with low rolling hills. | Reload week. |

Continue

| | | |
|---|---|---|
| 7 | Walk around with 45 pounds of additional load with weapon for 30 minutes at three to four miles per hour in an area with low rolling hills. | Review basic obstacles for 10 minutes. |
| 8 | Walk around with 50 pounds of additional load with weapon for 32 minutes at four miles per hour in an area with low rolling hills. | Continue weapon carriage with revised obstacles. |
| 9 | Walk around with 55 pounds of additional load with weapon for 34 minutes at four miles per hour in an area with low rolling hills. | |
| 10 | Walk around with 60 pounds of additional load with weapon for 30 minutes at four miles per hour in an area with low rolling hills. | Introduce steeper hills. |
| 11 | Walk around with 65 pounds of additional load with weapon for 33 minutes at four miles per hour in an area with low rolling hills. | Continue with steeper hills. |
| 12 | Battle simulation task for 40 minutes with 65 pounds of additional load. | |

Here is an eight-week program where the "theme" is provided for each training day; you can customize it exactly to your needs.

| Week # | Monday | Tuesday | Wednesday | Thursday | Friday | Saturday | Sunday |
|---|---|---|---|---|---|---|---|
| 1 | Strength Upper Body | Strength Lower Body | Aerobic Training | Strength Full Body | Rucking | Tempo Runs | Off |
| 2 | Strength Upper Body | Strength Lower Body | Aerobic Training | Strength Full Body | Rucking | Tempo Runs | Off |
| 3 | Strength Upper Body | Strength Lower Body | Aerobic Training | Strength Full Body | Rucking | Tempo Runs | Off |
| 4 | Strength Upper Body | Strength Lower Body | Aerobic Training | Strength Full Body | Rucking | Tempo Runs | Off |
| 5 | Strength Upper Body | Strength Lower Body | Aerobic Training | Strength Full Body | Rucking | Tempo Runs | Off |
| 6 | Strength Upper Body | Strength Lower Body | Aerobic Training | Strength Full Body | Rucking | Tempo Runs | Off |
| 7 | Strength Upper Body | Strength Lower Body | Aerobic Training | Strength Full Body | Rucking | Tempo Runs | Off |
| 8 Reload | Strength Upper Body | Strength Lower Body | Aerobic Training | Strength Full Body | Rucking | Tempo Runs | Off |

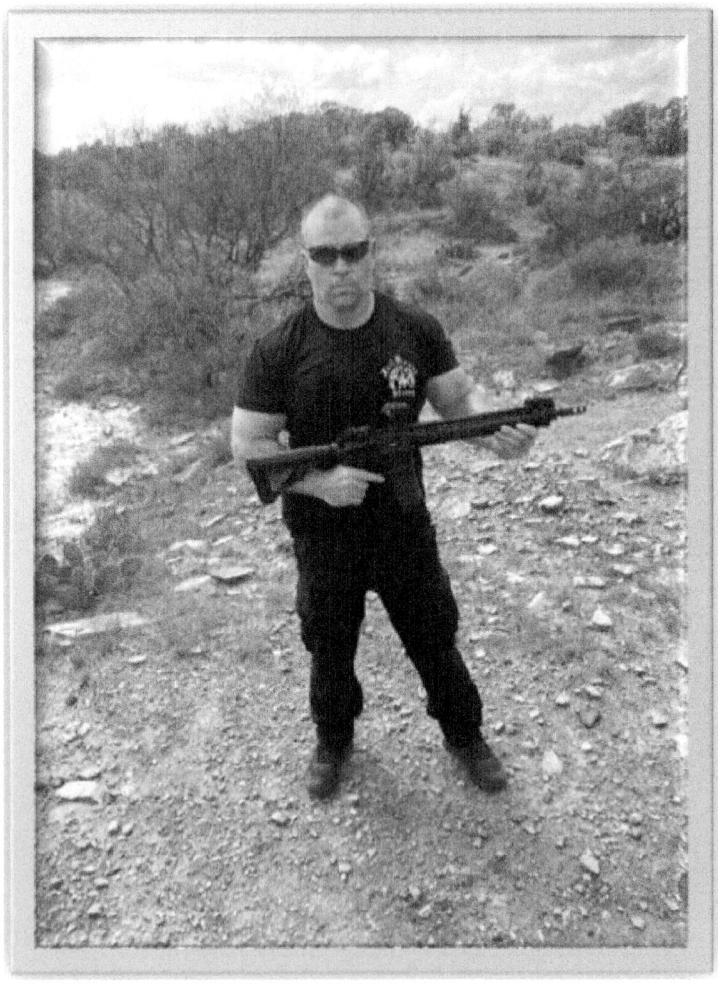

**Figure 9. Josh Bryant's boar hunting has been enhanced via rucking.**

## Final Thoughts

Knowledge is power!

With this knowledge, you now have the power to get ready for the upcoming assessment, prepare for the hunting trip, be a mother rucker as you tote around your toddler, or just get into great shape.

Remember, rucking is neither flashy nor boastful, but it can increase your strength, decrease your waistline, and make you move with greater aerobic capacity.

To use a metaphor from earlier, rucking is a well, not a fountain. It is time to explore its depths and make some rucking gains!

We are excited to hear more about your rucking journey. Connect with us on Instagram (@Jailhouse Strong), through YouTube (Jailhouse Strong), or by email (jailhousestrong@gmail.com).

Printed in Great Britain
by Amazon

18561444R00041